Cookbook: Flavors of West African Feasts

A Culinary Tapestry of Countries and Tribes

AFFUL CHRISTOPHER

DEDICATION

To the vibrant souls who embrace the art of West African cooking, This cookbook is lovingly dedicated to you, the culinary adventurers who seek the magic of West African flavors. It's a tribute to the countless kitchens where traditions are passed from generation to generation, and to the daring cooks who explore new tastes with zest. For those just beginning their journey, may this book be your guiding star through the aromatic world of West African cuisine. Here's to the joy of sharing meals, connecting hearts, and celebrating the diversity of this remarkable region.

INTRODUCTION

In a world where boundaries blur and cultures intermingle, few places exemplify the beauty of diversity like West Africa. Beyond its geographic expanse and breathtaking landscapes, West Africa is a tapestry of vibrant cultures, rich histories, and, perhaps most prominently, a culinary heritage that celebrates unity within diversity. In "West African Feasts: A Culinary Tapestry of Countries and Tribes," we invite you to embark on a culinary journey that transcends borders and delves deep into the heart of this dynamic region.

CONTENTS

CELEBRATING DIVERSITY ON THE PLATE

A Mosaic of Flavors and Traditions

Imagine sitting around a bustling West African table, where dishes brimming with diverse aromas and colors converge. This tableau, as diverse as the languages spoken and the stories shared, is a testament to the intricate mosaic of cultures that spans the countries and tribes of West Africa. From Nigeria's bustling markets to Senegal's coastal villages, from the lush landscapes of Ghana to the vibrant streets of Côte d'Ivoire, each region; has contributed to the rich gastronomic tapestry we celebrate.

Unity in Culinary Diversity

In West Africa, food is more than sustenance—it's a form of expression, a reflection of identity, and a bridge that connects generations. Every dish served is a living testament to the region's history, a tangible link to ancestors who lovingly passed down recipes, techniques, and culinary rituals. Yet, it's important to recognize that while individual dishes may hail from a particular tribe or country, they're embraced and enjoyed across borders, uniting West Africans in a shared culinary experience.

The Spirit of Sharing

West African feasts are a celebration of unity, and the concept of sharing goes beyond the mere exchange of food. It's an embodiment of community values, a way to strengthen bonds, and a means to create lasting memories. Whether it's a family gathering, a cultural celebration, or a communal event, the act of sharing a meal is a thread that weaves together the diverse fabrics of West African societies.

From Kitchens to Hearts: A Culinary Heritage

As we embark on this culinary expedition, we encourage you to not only discover the flavors that grace West African tables but also to immerse yourself in the stories behind each dish. The journey from the bustling markets to the kitchens where these feasts are crafted reveals the history, symbolism, and cultural nuances that have shaped West African cuisine.

A World of Flavor Awaits

Within the pages of "West African Feasts," you'll uncover the essence of each country's and tribe's culinary identity. From the bold spices of Nigeria to the coastal influences of Senegal, and from Ghana's heartwarming stews to the forest-inspired creations of Côte d'Ivoire, every chapter brings a new set of flavors and traditions to your plate.

A Shared Experience

"West African Feasts" celebrates not only the flavors of West Africa but also the spirit of togetherness that these feasts evoke. As you journey through the pages of this cookbook, we invite you to step into the shoes of West African families, to experience the camaraderie of communities, and to savor the joy of breaking bread with loved ones. Each recipe you'll find in "West African Feasts" is a portal to a world of flavors, a cultural journey, and an opportunity to partake in the heritage of West Africa. So, roll up your sleeves, open your heart to new tastes, and let the celebration of unity within diversity begin. As we bring these West African feasts to your kitchen, may you savor not only the flavors but also the stories, the histories, and the essence of a region that has beautifully woven its diversity onto every plate

CHAPTER 1
NIGERIA - FLAVORS OF THE NIGER DELTA

Welcome to the heart of Nigeria, where the Niger Delta region unfolds like a tapestry of flavors, cultures, and traditions. In this chapter, we invite you to explore the culinary treasures of Nigeria's diverse tribes, each contributing its own unique essence to the feasts that grace the tables of this dynamic country.

Culinary Kaleidoscope: Nigeria's Flavorful Diversity

Nigeria, often referred to as the "Giant of Africa," is a nation brimming with cultural diversity. The Niger Delta region, in particular, is a melting pot of culinary influences. From the Igbo people to the Ijaw, Urhobo, and Ogoni tribes, the region's culinary landscape is a testament to the unity within this diversity.

Jollof Rice: The Crown Jewel of Nigerian Cuisine

As you embark on your culinary journey through Nigeria's Niger Delta, you'll encounter a dish that reigns supreme on tables across the country: jollof rice. This fragrant creation, often accompanied by a vibrant array of vegetables and succulent meats, is the centerpiece of celebrations, marking joyous occasions with its vibrant colors and rich flavors. From the Ibibio tribe's spicy twist to the Itsekiri people's seafood-infused version, jollof rice encapsulates the essence of Nigeria's culinary prowess.

Egusi Soup and Other Delicacies: A Palate of Pleasure

Dive into the world of egusi soup, a beloved dish that showcases the Niger Delta's skillful blend of flavors and textures. Made from ground melon seeds, this soup is both hearty and nutritious, often accompanied by pounded yam or fufu. Explore the Okrika tribe's seafood delicacies, like pepper soup with fish or crab, and the Efik tribe's masterful use of spices in dishes that evoke warmth and comfort.

Savory Staples and Indigenous Ingredients
Nigerian cuisine draws heavily from indigenous ingredients, making use of yams, plantains, cassava, and a wide array of leafy vegetables. The Urhobo tribe's starch-based cuisine, featuring pounded yam and banga soup, highlights the region's affinity for hearty and satisfying dishes. Additionally, the Isoko tribe's creative use of cocoyam and periwinkle adds a unique dimension to the culinary tapestry.

Ijaw Delights: Seafood and Coconut Creations
As you explore the Ijaw tribe's cuisine, you'll be transported to the coastal landscapes of the Niger Delta. Seafood takes center stage in dishes like boli and fish pepper soup, capturing the essence of the region's proximity to the ocean. The Ijaw people's ingenious use of coconut in soups and stews adds a tropical twist to their culinary repertoire.

Cultural Traditions and Culinary Expressions
Nigeria's Niger Delta is not only a region of diverse flavors but also a canvas for cultural expressions. The Ogba tribe's love for roasted plantains and palm wine reflects a simple yet profound connection to the land. As you delve into the cuisine, you'll gain insight into the rituals and customs that shape the way Niger Delta tribes celebrate, bond, and express their identities.

Beyond the Plate: Community and Togetherness
Nigerian feasts are a reflection of the region's strong sense of community. The act of sharing a meal transcends mere sustenance—it's a gesture of love, a symbol of unity, and a testament to the bonds that tie families and communities together. As you explore the flavors of the Niger Delta, you'll come to appreciate how every dish carries within it the spirit of togetherness and the joy of coming together around a communal table.

Bringing the Feast to Your Kitchen

Throughout this chapter, you'll find authentic recipes that capture the essence of Nigeria's Niger Delta. From jollof rice to egusi soup, each recipe comes with step-by-step instructions and insights into the cultural significance of the dish. By recreating these flavors in your own kitchen, you'll not only savor the richness of the Niger Delta but also embrace the spirit of unity that these feasts symbolize.

Embrace the warmth, diversity, and unity of Nigeria's Niger Delta as you journey through its culinary treasures. Each recipe is an invitation to experience the flavors, traditions, and stories that shape the region's vibrant tapestry. So, roll up your sleeves, let your senses guide you, and savor the richness of Nigeria's culinary heritage—one dish at a time.

CHAPTER 2
SENEGAL - COASTAL TREASURES

Welcome to the sun-kissed shores of Senegal, where the gentle rhythm of the waves echoes in the flavors of the cuisine. In this chapter, we invite you to explore the vibrant culinary tapestry of Senegal, a nation where coastal influences blend seamlessly with cultural traditions to create dishes that celebrate the bounty of both land and sea.

The Melting Pot of Senegalese Cuisine

Senegal's coastal location has given rise to a cuisine that harmoniously marries indigenous flavors with global influences. From the Wolof tribe to the Serer and Fula people, the diversity of Senegal's ethnic groups is beautifully mirrored in its culinary traditions, creating a kaleidoscope of flavors that tantalize the palate.

Thieboudienne: A Feast of the Coast

As you embark on your culinary journey through Senegal, you'll encounter the crown jewel of Senegalese cuisine: thieboudienne. This flavorful one-pot dish is a symphony of flavors, combining rice, fish, and an array of vegetables, all simmered in a tomato-based sauce. Thieboudienne reflects the coastal essence of Senegal, capturing the flavors of the sea and the bounty of the land in a single dish.

Seafood Extravaganza: A Tribute to the Ocean

Senegal's proximity to the Atlantic Ocean infuses its cuisine with an abundance of seafood delights. From the rich seafood stews enjoyed by the Wolof tribe to the grilled fish cherished by the Fula people, Senegal's culinary identity is intimately linked to the treasures of the sea. Explore dishes like yassa poisson, where fish is marinated in tangy lemon and onion sauce, and let the flavors transport you to Senegal's sun-drenched coastlines.

Benechin and the Art of Rice Variations

Rice is a staple of Senegalese cuisine, often taking center stage in dishes that vary from region to region. Benechin, a dish that originated from the Wolof tribe, showcases Senegal's ability to transform simple ingredients into a symphony of taste. The combination of rice, vegetables, and protein creates a harmonious melody of flavors that resonates with every bite.

Sweet and Spicy: Senegalese Flavors

Unveiled Senegalese cuisine embraces a delightful juxtaposition of sweet and spicy notes, as exemplified by dishes like mafé. This peanut stew, enjoyed by various tribes, brings together tender meat and hearty vegetables in a velvety sauce enriched with ground peanuts. The balance of flavors is a testament to Senegal's culinary finesse and its ability to create dishes that delight the senses.

Street Food Culture: Senegal's Culinary Vibrancy

Explore the vibrant street food culture of Senegal, where the bustling markets are alive with the aromas of savory snacks and hearty meals. Sink your teeth into bissap, a hibiscus-infused drink enjoyed throughout Senegal, and discover the addictive flavors of accara, deep-fried black-eyed pea fritters. Senegal's street food scene captures the vivacity of the nation's culinary heritage in every bite.

Preserving Traditions Through Food

Senegal's culinary traditions are intrinsically tied to its cultural heritage. The Serer tribe's emphasis on local ingredients and natural flavors reflects the respect for the land and its offerings. The Fula people's use of millet in dishes like thiakry showcases the resourcefulness and creativity that define Senegal's cuisine.

Culinary Reflections: From Ocean to Plate

Senegalese feasts are not just about indulging the palate; they're an embodiment of culture, unity, and the joy of sharing a meal. Whether it's celebrating family milestones or coming together during festivals, Senegal's cuisine is a testament to the role that food plays in strengthening bonds and nurturing relationships.

Bringing Senegal's Coastal Treasures to Your Table

Throughout this chapter, you'll discover authentic recipes that capture the essence of Senegal's coastal cuisine. From thieboudienne to yassa poisson, each recipe is an invitation to experience the vibrant flavors and cultural nuances that shape Senegal's culinary identity. By recreating these dishes in your own kitchen, you'll be transported to Senegal's sun-drenched shores, where the aroma of the ocean mingles with the rich tapestry of flavors that define this coastal paradise.

CHAPTER 3
GHANA - AKAN DELIGHTS

Step into the heart of Ghana, a land where Akan traditions and culinary treasures intertwine to create a symphony of flavors that celebrate community, heritage, and the vibrant spirit of West Africa. In this chapter, we invite you to explore the rich tapestry of Akan cuisine, where dishes cherished by the Ashanti, Fante, Akuapem, and other tribes reflect the essence of Ghana's culinary identity.

Akan Culture: The Foundation of Ghana's Culinary Landscape
Ghana's Akan tribes are at the core of the nation's cultural fabric, and their culinary traditions hold a special place in the hearts and stomachs of Ghanaians. From the Ashanti people's grand feasts to the Fante tribe's coastal influences, Akan cuisine is a mirror that reflects the diversity and unity within the country's culinary landscape.

Comfort and Celebration: The Soulful Essence of Akan Dishes
At the heart of Akan cuisine lies a celebration of tradition, community, and the nurturing power of food. Dishes like fufu and light soups encapsulate the idea of comfort and togetherness, nourishing both body and soul. Whether it's the Akuapem tribe's abenkwan or the Nzema people's wakye, Akan dishes evoke a sense of belonging and celebration.

Fufu: An Akan Culinary Icon
Fufu is not just a dish; it's a cultural emblem that embodies the essence of Akan cuisine. The rhythmic pounding of yam, plantains, or cassava to create the smooth, starchy fufu reflects the labor of love that goes into every meal. Whether paired with okra soup, palm nut soup, or groundnut soup, fufu is the ultimate expression of Akan culinary artistry.

Plantains and Hearty Stews: A Perfect Harmony

Plantains, a versatile ingredient, find their way into many Akan dishes, adding sweetness and substance to meals. Discover the Ashanti people's sumptuous eto and nkotomire stew, where the delicate balance of flavors showcases the region's culinary finesse. Explore the Akuapem tribe's love for banku and okra soup, a cherished combination that brings comfort and satisfaction.

Seafood and Salt: A Coastal Connection

The Fante tribe's coastal location infuses their cuisine with the flavors of the ocean. Dishes like fante fante and fisherman's stew celebrate the bounty of the sea, while the Akan tradition of using salt as a symbol of hospitality and friendship is woven into the very fabric of these dishes. Coastal influences meld seamlessly with Akan traditions, creating flavors that evoke the rhythm of the waves.

Sweets and Treats: Akan Indulgences

Satisfy your sweet tooth with Akan desserts that reflect the tribe's creativity and passion for flavor. The Akuapem people's akatse, a deep-fried corn dough, and the Ashanti tribe's bofrot, a popular street food, showcase the joy of indulging in treats that are both comforting and delectable.

The Role of Akan Cuisine in Daily Life

In Akan culture, food is more than sustenance—it's a symbol of respect, unity, and shared experiences. The Ashanti people's ritual of pouring libations and sharing meals during important gatherings illustrates the role that food plays in honoring ancestors and fostering connections. Akan cuisine is a way of life that binds families, strengthens friendships, and celebrates the bonds that tie communities together.

Honoring Ancestry Through Food

Akan feasts are an embodiment of the spirit of unity and respect for ancestry. The Adinkra symbols that grace Akan dishes carry deeper meanings that honor traditions, values, and the importance of community. From the Sankofa symbol that signifies the importance of learning from the past to the Nyame Dua, the sacred tree of God, each symbol is a reminder of the rich cultural heritage that underpins Akan cuisine.

Bringing Akan Delights to Your Table

Throughout this chapter, you'll uncover a treasure trove of authentic Akan recipes that embody the flavors and stories of Ghana. From fufu to eto, each dish comes with step-by-step instructions and insights into the cultural significance behind it. By recreating these dishes in your own kitchen, you'll not only savor the richness of Akan cuisine but also embrace the spirit of unity, tradition, and community that these feasts symbolize.

Step into the world of Akan delights, where each recipe is an invitation to experience the flavors, traditions, and stories that shape Ghana's vibrant culinary heritage. As you savor the richness of Akan cuisine, you'll be transported to the heart of Ghana—a place where food is more than nourishment; it's a celebration of culture, a reflection of community, and a tribute to the spirit of unity that binds the Akan people together.

CHAPTER 4
CÔTE D'IVOIRE - FOREST FLAVORS

Enter the enchanting world of Côte d'Ivoire, where the lush forests and vibrant cultures come together to create a culinary tapestry that reflects the bounties of the land and the diversity of its people. In this chapter, we invite you to explore the flavors of Côte d'Ivoire, a country where the cuisine is deeply rooted in the forests, traditions, and vibrant spirit of West Africa.

A Glimpse into Côte d'Ivoire's Culinary Mosaic

Côte d'Ivoire, often referred to as the "Ivory Coast," is a country that boasts a rich cultural and ethnic diversity. The flavors of its cuisine reflect the influences of the Baoulé, Bété, Senufo, and other tribes that have shaped its culinary identity. As we journey through Côte d'Ivoire's forest flavors, you'll discover dishes that celebrate the region's natural bounty and cultural heritage.

Palm Trees and Placali: Celebrating the Land's Offerings

Central to Côte d'Ivoire's culinary landscape is the palm tree, a symbol of abundance and sustenance. Placali, a fermented cassava dish enjoyed by the Bété tribe, showcases the resourcefulness of the Ivorian people. Delve into the Senufo tribe's use of millet and sorghum in dishes like tô and discover how these staple foods nourish both body and soul.

Sauce Kôkô: The Essence of Ivorian Comfort

One of Côte d'Ivoire's signature dishes, sauce kôkô, epitomizes the harmony between forest ingredients and cultural heritage. This spinach stew, often paired with fish or meat, is enjoyed by various tribes and carries the flavors of the land within its savory depths. As you savor each spoonful of sauce kôkô, you'll experience the essence of Ivorian comfort and the love that goes into preparing every meal.

Cassava and Yams: Ivorian Staples

Cassava and yams are staples in Ivorian cuisine, forming the basis of many dishes enjoyed across the country. From the Yacouba tribe's use of cassava in dishes like foutou to the Akwiwé people's creative yam preparations, these tubers are not just ingredients but cultural symbols that embody the Ivorian way of life.

Bitterleaf Soup and Cultural Expressions

The Bété tribe's bitterleaf soup stands as a testament to Côte d'Ivoire's connection to its forests. Made from the leaves of the bitterleaf plant, this soup encapsulates the Ivorian people's skill in utilizing the land's offerings. As you explore the flavors of this dish and others like it, you'll gain insight into the cultural expressions and culinary traditions that define the region.

Variety in Ivorian Cuisine: A Feast of Vegetables

Ivorian cuisine celebrates the diversity of vegetables that thrive in the region's fertile soils. The Dan tribe's use of eggplant in dishes like sauce djoumblé highlights the Ivorian people's ability to transform simple ingredients into vibrant and flavorful creations. Dive into the array of vegetables used in Ivorian cuisine, and you'll uncover a world of color, taste, and nutritional richness.

Crafting Culinary Traditions Through Generations

Côte d'Ivoire's culinary traditions are an integral part of family life, passed down from generation to generation. The region's feasts are not just meals; they're stories, traditions, and a reflection of the Ivorian people's respect for their heritage. The art of storytelling is woven into each dish, creating a tapestry that binds families and communities together.

Balancing Flavors: Sweet and Savory Harmonies

Ivorian cuisine embraces the balance between sweet and savory, creating dishes that dance on the palate. The Attié tribe's use of honey in dishes like aloko adds a touch of sweetness to complement the savory flavors of the cuisine. Discover how Ivorian culinary artists harmonize these flavors to create dishes that captivate the senses.

Nurturing Connections Through Food

Ivorian feasts go beyond the table; they're a celebration of life, community, and the bonds that tie people together. The joy of gathering around a meal with loved ones and sharing stories reflects the Ivorian people's deep appreciation for togetherness and unity.

Bringing Forest Flavors to Your Table

Throughout this chapter, you'll uncover a diverse range of authentic Ivorian recipes that embody the forest flavors and cultural richness of Côte d'Ivoire. From sauce kôkô to bitterleaf soup, each dish comes with step-by-step instructions and insights into the cultural significance behind it. By recreating these dishes in your own kitchen, you'll not only savor the essence of Côte d'Ivoire's cuisine but also experience the deep connection to the land and culture that these feasts represent. Step into the world of Ivorian forest flavors, where each recipe is an invitation to explore the tastes, traditions, and stories that shape Côte d'Ivoire's culinary tapestry. As you savor the richness of Ivorian cuisine, you'll be transported to the heart of the forests—a place where food is more than nourishment; it's a celebration of nature, culture, and the unity that binds the Ivorian people together.

CHAPTER 5
LIBERIA - PEPPER SOUP AND PALAVA

Welcome to the captivating world of Liberia, a country that tells its story through the bold flavors and vibrant colors of its cuisine. In this chapter, we invite you to explore the culinary traditions of Liberia, where dishes like pepper soup and palava are a testament to the resilience, warmth, and diverse heritage of the Liberian people.

Unveiling Liberia's Culinary Mosaic

Liberia, known as the "Land of the Free," is a nation that echoes the stories of its people through its food. The flavors of its cuisine reflect the harmonious blend of tribes and cultures that form the foundation of Liberian identity. From the Vai people's pepper soup to the Bassa tribe's palava, Liberia's culinary traditions celebrate both unity and diversity.

Pepper Soup: A Liberian Comfort Classic

As you step into Liberia's culinary landscape, you'll encounter a dish that warms the heart and soothes the soul: pepper soup. This beloved Liberian classic, enjoyed by various tribes, brings together tender meats, hearty vegetables, and a medley of aromatic spices that create a symphony of flavors. Whether it's fish, chicken, or goat, pepper soup reflects the Liberian spirit of comfort and hospitality.

Palava: A Melody of Flavors

Palava, often prepared with greens, meat, and palm oil, is a dish that embodies the essence of Liberian cuisine. The Bassa tribe's version, featuring cassava leaves and smoked fish, captures the flavors of the land and the sea. Palava is more than just a dish; it's a culinary melody that harmonizes tradition, taste, and a deep connection to the environment.

Rice: The Heartbeat of Liberian Meals

Rice holds a special place in Liberian hearts and kitchens. The Fulani tribe's benachin, a one-pot rice and fish creation, is a testament to the importance of rice in Liberian cuisine. Whether it's served with pepper soup or paired with palava, rice unites Liberians in a shared love for this staple food.

Leafy Greens and Indigenous Ingredients

Liberian cuisine is abundant with leafy greens and indigenous ingredients that reflect the country's natural wealth. The Gio tribe's use of potato greens and the Kpelle people's incorporation of cassava leaves highlight the culinary creativity that thrives in Liberia's kitchens. These ingredients not only nourish the body but also celebrate the land's offerings.

Community and Cuisine: The Liberian Way

Liberia's feasts are a celebration of unity and togetherness, reflecting the deep sense of community that defines its people. The Bassa people's tradition of sharing palava with extended family and friends showcases the role of food in fostering connections and strengthening bonds.

Spices and Stories: Flavorful Conversations

Liberian cuisine is a vehicle for storytelling, with flavors that evoke memories and experiences. The use of spices, like ginger, garlic, and hot peppers, infuses each dish with depth and character. The Kru tribe's use of hot peppers in dishes like pepper soup reflects the Liberian people's zest for life and their ability to turn meals into vibrant conversations.

Culinary Wisdom and Generational Ties

Liberian culinary traditions are passed down from generation to generation, preserving not only flavors but also family connections. The wisdom shared between grandparents and grandchildren during cooking sessions creates a bridge between the past and the present, ensuring that Liberian heritage is savored with every bite.

Harmony in Diversity: A Liberian Feast

Liberia's feasts are a reflection of the nation's diverse cultural landscape. The blending of Bassa, Kpelle, Gio, and other tribes' flavors in a single meal represents the unity that arises from diversity. Liberian cuisine is a testament to the fact that despite differences, the love for food brings people together in harmony.

Bringing Liberia's Culinary Melodies to Your Table

Throughout this chapter, you'll uncover a treasure trove of authentic Liberian recipes that embody the flavors and stories of the country. From pepper soup to palava, each dish comes with step-by-step instructions and insights into the cultural significance behind it. By recreating these dishes in your own kitchen, you'll not only savor the richness of Liberian cuisine but also embrace the spirit of community, storytelling, and unity that these feasts symbolize.

Step into the world of Liberian pepper soup and palava, where each recipe is an invitation to experience the flavors, traditions, and stories that shape Liberia's vibrant culinary heritage. As you savor the richness of Liberian cuisine, you'll be transported to the heart of the country— a place where food is more than nourishment; it's a celebration of culture, a reflection of community, and a tribute to the spirit of unity that binds the Liberian people together.

CHAPTER 6
MALI - SAHARAN FLAVORS

Welcome to the expansive landscapes of Mali, where the golden sands of the Sahara Desert meet the rich traditions and flavors of West African cuisine. In this chapter, we invite you to explore the culinary treasures of Mali, a country where Saharan influences are beautifully woven into dishes that tell stories of resilience, culture, and the vibrant spirit of the desert.

Mali's Culinary Journey: A Tale of Diversity

Mali, often referred to as the "Gateway to the Sahara," is a nation that embraces its diverse cultures and traditions. The flavors of its cuisine reflect the influences of the Bambara, Tuareg, Soninke, and other tribes that contribute to Mali's vibrant tapestry. From the banks of the Niger River to the edges of the desert, Mali's culinary traditions celebrate both unity and distinctiveness.

The Sahara on a Plate: Fulfilling Meals in Harsh Landscapes

As you embark on your culinary journey through Mali, you'll discover dishes that have stood the test of time and are cherished in the midst of the desert's challenges. Mafé, a peanut-based stew enjoyed by the Bambara tribe, exemplifies Mali's ability to transform humble ingredients into a feast that nourishes both body and soul. This dish is a testament to the culinary creativity born out of necessity in the desert environment.

Couscous and Comfort: Tuareg Culinary Artistry

Couscous, a staple of Saharan cuisine, takes center stage in Mali's culinary offerings. The Tuareg people's mastery of couscous preparation is evident in dishes like tefou, where the semolina pearls are paired with meat and vegetables. These creations capture the essence of the desert, reflecting the Tuareg people's ability to transform simple ingredients into comfort food that resonates with the heart.

Savory Delicacies from the Sahel: A Taste of Mali

The Sahel region of Mali is known for its rich culinary heritage, with dishes that pay homage to both the desert and the Sahel's fertile lands. Discover the Songhai tribe's use of millet in dishes like tô, a staple food that sustains communities across the region. Explore Mali's love for okra and explore dishes that bridge the gap between land and desert.

African Rice and Cultural Symbols

Rice holds cultural significance in Mali, symbolizing unity, abundance, and the joy of sharing a meal. The Bambara people's use of rice in dishes like riz gras reflects Mali's ability to infuse everyday ingredients with flavors that delight and satisfy. The act of preparing and sharing rice dishes is a reflection of Mali's values, creating a sense of community and togetherness.

Dunes and Desert Dishes: Navigating Flavorful Landscapes

Mali's cuisine captures the essence of the desert's diverse landscapes, from the shifting dunes to the vibrant oases. The Dogon people's use of millet and vegetables in dishes like toh and takouya showcases the delicate balance between sustenance and flavor that defines Saharan cuisine. These dishes embody the resourcefulness and ingenuity that arise from living in challenging environments.

Culinary Traditions: Nurturing Identity

Mali's culinary traditions are a reflection of the people's deep connection to their land, history, and traditions. The Bambara people's use of tamarind and baobab leaves in dishes like kapoké highlights the way Mali's cuisine weaves cultural heritage into every bite. Each dish is a tribute to the stories passed down through generations, nurturing the sense of identity that binds communities together.

Saharan Spice and Sahel Soul: Harmonizing Flavors

Mali's cuisine is a symphony of flavors that harmonize spices, vegetables, and proteins in a delicate dance of taste. The Soninke people's use of onions, tomatoes, and chili peppers in dishes like jollof rice showcases Mali's ability to create dishes that capture the vibrancy of the Sahel. The balance of flavors reflects Mali's culinary finesse and its ability to create meals that resonate with the senses.

Food as a Cultural Bridge

In Mali, food is a bridge that connects people, traditions, and landscapes. The Soninke tribe's tradition of sharing food during important events symbolizes the way Mali's cuisine fosters connections and celebrations. Meals are more than sustenance; they're an expression of culture, a reflection of community, and a testament to the enduring spirit of the Sahel.

Bringing Saharan Flavors to Your Table

Throughout this chapter, you'll uncover authentic recipes that capture the essence of Mali's Saharan cuisine. From mafé to tefou, each dish comes with step-by-step instructions and insights into the cultural significance of the ingredients used. By recreating these dishes in your own kitchen, you'll not only savor the richness of Mali's culinary heritage but also embrace the spirit of resourcefulness, culture, and unity that these feasts symbolize. Step into the world of Mali's Saharan flavors, where each recipe is an invitation to experience the tastes, traditions, and stories that shape the country's vibrant culinary tapestry. As you savor the richness of Mali's cuisine, you'll be transported to the heart of the Sahara—a place where food is more than nourishment; it's a celebration of resilience, culture, and the unity that binds the Malian people together.

CHAPTER 7
THE GAMBIA - MANDINKA HERITAGE

Welcome to The Gambia, a land where the mighty Gambia River winds through lush landscapes and vibrant cultures. In this chapter, we invite you to explore the culinary treasures of The Gambia, a country where Mandinka traditions and flavors come alive, celebrating the richness of the land and the enduring spirit of its people.

A Glimpse into Mandinka Culture

The Gambia, often referred to as the "Smiling Coast of Africa," is a nation that embraces its cultural diversity. The flavors of its cuisine reflect the influences of the Mandinka people, whose traditions and heritage form an integral part of Gambian identity. From the banks of the river to the heart of the villages, Gambian culinary traditions tell stories of unity and belonging.

Mandinka Heritage on the Plate: Groundnut Stew

As you embark on your culinary journey through The Gambia, you'll encounter a dish that is beloved by the Mandinka people and revered across the country: groundnut stew. This rich, peanut-based concoction is a hallmark of Gambian cuisine, capturing the essence of the land and its people. The Mandinka people's skillful use of peanuts, vegetables, and proteins in dishes like domoda reflects their ability to transform simple ingredients into culinary masterpieces.

Rice and Grains: A Gambian Staple

Rice and grains are at the heart of Gambian meals, showcasing the Mandinka people's ingenuity in creating nourishing and flavorful dishes. From the traditional rice and millet porridge known as benachin to the Mandinka people's use of couscous in dishes like garawol, the Gambia's culinary landscape is a celebration of the land's bounty and the people's resourcefulness.

Baobab Delicacies: A Tangy Twist

Baobab fruit holds a special place in Gambian cuisine, adding a tangy twist to dishes and beverages. The Mandinka people's use of baobab in dishes like baobab juice reflects the Gambia's connection to its natural resources. Explore how baobab is incorporated into the cuisine, infusing it with a unique flavor that mirrors the Gambian spirit.

Fish and the River's Bounty

The Gambia River is the lifeblood of the nation, providing a rich source of fish that features prominently in Gambian cuisine. The Mandinka people's mastery of fish preparation is evident in dishes like benachin with fish, where the river's bounty is honored through flavorful combinations. The Gambia's connection to the river is not only sustenance but also a reflection of the nation's culture and livelihood.

Flavors of Nature: Palm Wine and Tamarind

Gambian cuisine often draws inspiration from the natural world, incorporating ingredients like palm wine and tamarind to create unique and delightful flavors. The Mandinka people's use of palm wine in dishes like benachin with palm wine showcases the harmony between nature and culinary artistry. Dive into the flavors of these ingredients and uncover how they contribute to the Gambian culinary experience.

Family, Food, and Festivals

Gambian feasts are a celebration of life's milestones and the bonds that tie families and communities together. The Mandinka people's tradition of sharing meals during important events and festivals reflects the role that food plays in fostering connections and creating cherished memories. In Gambian culture, the act of sharing a meal is a reflection of love, unity, and the joy of coming together.

Culinary Storytelling and Tradition

Mandinka culinary traditions are an integral part of Gambian culture, reflecting the values, stories, and heritage of the people. The Gambia's love for spicy flavors, as seen in dishes like benachin, is a testament to the way food carries the essence of tradition and memory. Each dish is a chapter in the story of the Gambia, connecting past and present through the art of cooking.

Harmony in the Kitchen: Mandinka Culinary Craftsmanship

The Mandinka people's culinary expertise is evident in the way they balance flavors and ingredients to create dishes that resonate with the palate. The use of spices, herbs, and seasonings in dishes like benachin with chicken reflects the Gambian ability to turn meals into harmonious and flavorful experiences.

Preserving Heritage Through Food

In The Gambia, food is a vessel for cultural preservation, allowing traditions to be passed down through generations. The Mandinka people's commitment to preserving their culinary heritage ensures that the flavors and stories of the Gambia's past remain alive in every dish.

Bringing Mandinka Heritage to Your Table

Throughout this chapter, you'll discover authentic recipes that capture the essence of the Gambia's Mandinka cuisine. From groundnut stew to benachin, each dish comes with step-by-step instructions and insights into the cultural significance behind it. By recreating these dishes in your own kitchen, you'll not only savor the richness of Gambian cuisine but also embrace the spirit of Mandinka heritage, unity, and celebration that these feasts symbolize.

Step into the world of Mandinka heritage, where each recipe is an invitation to experience the flavors, traditions, and stories that shape the Gambia's vibrant culinary tapestry. As you savor the richness of Gambian cuisine, you'll be transported to the heart of the country—a place where food is more than nourishment; it's a celebration of culture, a reflection of community, and a tribute to the enduring spirit of the Gambian people.

CHAPTER 8
SIERRA LEONE - KRIO CREATIONS

Step into the vibrant world of Sierra Leone, a country where cultures converge to create a unique culinary experience known as Krio cuisine. In this chapter, we invite you to explore the flavors of Sierra Leone, where Krio creations celebrate the fusion of cultures, the bounties of the land, and the resilient spirit of its people.

Embracing Krio Culture

Sierra Leone is a nation that embodies diversity, and its cuisine reflects the melting pot of cultures that have come together to shape its identity. The Krio people, descendants of freed slaves and liberated Africans, have enriched Sierra Leone's cultural tapestry and cuisine with their unique fusion of African, European, and Caribbean influences.

Krio Delicacies: A Culinary Fusion

As you embark on your culinary journey through Sierra Leone, you'll encounter Krio creations that capture the essence of this cultural fusion. One such dish is jollof rice, a popular West African rice dish that has found a special place in Krio cuisine. The Krio people's adaptation of jollof rice is a symbol of their ability to combine diverse flavors to create something truly exceptional.

Rice and the Krio Kitchen

Rice is a cornerstone of Sierra Leonean cuisine, and Krio kitchens are no exception. From the Krio people's version of fried rice to the incorporation of seafood and vegetables, rice dishes are a canvas for creativity in Krio culinary artistry. These dishes reflect the Krio people's knack for blending cultural elements to craft unique flavors.

The Essence of Krio Cuisine: Cassava Leaves

Cassava leaves hold a special place in Krio cuisine, representing the connection to the land and the celebration of shared heritage. The Krio people's preparation of cassava leaves with palm oil, often enjoyed with rice or foofoo, showcases their ability to transform simple ingredients into dishes that embody the spirit of Sierra Leone.

Seafood and the Atlantic Influence

Sierra Leone's coastal location infuses its cuisine with a rich variety of seafood. The Krio people's mastery of seafood preparation is evident in dishes like pepper soup with fish, which reflects the Atlantic's influence on the culinary landscape. Seafood dishes in Krio cuisine are not just meals; they're an ode to the ocean's bounty and the Krio people's relationship with their environment.

Flavors from Afar: The Influence of Caribbean Cuisine

The Krio people's roots in the Caribbean have left a distinct mark on Sierra Leonean cuisine. Dishes like fried plantains and akara, a deep-fried bean cake, showcase the Caribbean influences that have merged seamlessly with Sierra Leonean flavors. These creations celebrate the resilience of the Krio people and the way their culinary journey has come full circle.

Krio Celebrations: Food as a Symbol of Unity

In Krio culture, food is more than sustenance; it's a symbol of unity, identity, and celebration. Krio celebrations are characterized by feasts that bring families, friends, and communities together. The Krio people's tradition of sharing meals during events like naming ceremonies and weddings reflects the importance of food in fostering connections and honoring traditions.

Culinary Connections: Krio Diaspora

The Krio diaspora has spread Krio cuisine and culture to various parts of the world, creating a sense of belonging and nostalgia for those who carry Sierra Leone in their hearts. The Krio people's ability to preserve their culinary traditions in different corners of the globe is a testament to the enduring legacy of their heritage.

Krio Craftsmanship: Flavorful Artistry

Krio cuisine is a testament to the Krio people's culinary craftsmanship, as they skillfully blend ingredients, flavors, and techniques to create dishes that tell stories of history, culture, and unity. The use of spices like ginger, cloves, and nutmeg in dishes like kanya and poyo chicken exemplifies the Krio people's ability to craft flavors that are both rich and nuanced.

Preserving Tradition Through Food

Krio cuisine serves as a vessel for preserving Sierra Leonean heritage and passing it down to future generations. The Krio people's commitment to keeping their culinary traditions alive ensures that the flavors, stories, and values of Sierra Leone are celebrated with every bite.

Bringing Krio Creations to Your Table

Throughout this chapter, you'll uncover a treasure trove of authentic Krio recipes that embody the flavors and stories of Sierra Leone. From jollof rice to cassava leaves, each dish comes with step-by-step instructions and insights into the cultural significance behind it. By recreating these dishes in your own kitchen, you'll not only savor the richness of Sierra Leonean cuisine but also embrace the spirit of Krio heritage, diversity, and unity that these feasts symbolize.

Step into the world of Krio creations, where each recipe is an invitation to experience the flavors, traditions, and stories that shape Sierra Leone's vibrant culinary tapestry. As you savor the richness of Sierra Leonean cuisine, you'll be transported to the heart of the country—a place where food is more than nourishment; it's a celebration of culture, a reflection of community, and a tribute to the enduring spirit of the Sierra Leonean people.

CHAPTER 9
BURKINA FASO - SAVANNA STAPLES

Welcome to the captivating landscapes of Burkina Faso, where the vast savannas meet the rich culinary traditions of West Africa. In this chapter, we invite you to explore the flavors of Burkina Faso, where savanna staples celebrate the harmony between the land, its people, and the cultural tapestry that defines this nation.

Journeying Through Burkina Faso's Savannas
Burkina Faso, often referred to as the "Land of Upright People," is a nation that embraces the rhythms of its savannas and the diversity of its ethnic groups. The flavors of its cuisine reflect the influences of the Mossi, Fulani, Bwa, and other tribes that contribute to Burkina Faso's rich cultural mosaic. From the rural villages to the bustling cities, Burkina Faso's culinary traditions celebrate both tradition and innovation.

Millets and Sorghum: Burkina Faso's Culinary Cornerstones
As you embark on your culinary journey through Burkina Faso, you'll discover the significance of millets and sorghum in the nation's cuisine. These hearty grains are not just ingredients; they're symbols of resilience and adaptability in the face of challenging landscapes. The Mossi people's use of millet in dishes like tô, a staple food enjoyed with sauces, reflects the way these grains sustain communities and tell stories of sustenance.

Sauce and Community: The Essence of Burkina Faso's Cuisine
Sauces play a central role in Burkina Faso's culinary culture, transforming simple ingredients into flavorful and nourishing dishes. The Fulani people's use of okra in dishes like riz sauce gombo highlights the way sauces bring people together and create a sense of belonging. In Burkina Faso, a meal is not just a plate; it's a communal experience that reflects the bonds of family, friends, and culture.

Millet Beer and Cultural Traditions

Burkina Faso's cuisine extends beyond the plate to include beverages that are deeply woven into the fabric of daily life. The Bwa people's millet beer, known as dolo, is a testament to the way beverages serve as cultural symbols and mediums for storytelling. Discover how these beverages connect people, traditions, and the land in a flavorful expression of Burkina Faso's spirit.

Fulani Heritage: Dairy Delights

The Fulani people's nomadic lifestyle has shaped their culinary traditions, resulting in a unique emphasis on dairy products. Dishes like fulfulde milk porridge and nono showcase the Fulani people's mastery of dairy preparation. These creations celebrate Burkina Faso's pastoral landscapes and the deep connection between the Fulani people and their herds.

Nuts and Flavorful Foundations

Nuts, such as peanuts and shea nuts, hold a special place in Burkina Faso's cuisine, adding depth and flavor to a variety of dishes. The Bwa people's use of shea nuts in dishes like soup reveals the culinary versatility of these ingredients and their ability to enhance flavors in unexpected ways.

Savanna Celebrations: Rituals of Joy

In Burkina Faso, food is an integral part of celebrations, rituals, and ceremonies. The Mossi people's tradition of sharing meals during important events, such as weddings and funerals, showcases the role of food in honoring traditions and fostering connections. Each bite is a testament to the importance of these rituals in Burkina Faso's cultural fabric.

Culinary Artistry and Expression

Burkina Faso's cuisine is a canvas for creativity, where ingredients are transformed into flavorful masterpieces. The Mossi people's use of baobab leaves in dishes like sauce feuilles de baobab exemplifies the artistry that goes into crafting meals that are not only delicious but also visually appealing.

Unity Through Food: A Burkina Faso Feast

Burkina Faso's feasts are a reflection of the unity and togetherness that define its people. The Mossi people's tradition of sharing meals in a communal setting showcases the way food brings people together, fosters conversations, and strengthens the bonds of community.

Passing Down Tradition: The Role of Elders

In Burkina Faso, culinary traditions are preserved through the wisdom of elders, who pass down recipes, techniques, and stories to younger generations. The Bwa people's use of traditional cooking methods in dishes like binga is a testament to the enduring legacy of Burkina Faso's culinary heritage.

Bringing Savanna Staples to Your Table

Throughout this chapter, you'll uncover a treasure trove of authentic recipes that embody the flavors and stories of Burkina Faso's savanna cuisine. From tô to dolo, each dish comes with step-by-step instructions and insights into the cultural significance behind it. By recreating these dishes in your own kitchen, you'll not only savor the richness of Burkina Faso's culinary heritage but also embrace the spirit of unity, resilience, and culture that these feasts symbolize.

Step into the world of Burkina Faso's savanna staples, where each recipe is an invitation to experience the flavors, traditions, and stories that shape the nation's vibrant culinary tapestry. As you savor the richness of Burkina Faso's cuisine, you'll be transported to the heart of the savannas—a place where food is more than nourishment; it's a celebration of culture, a reflection of community, and a tribute to the enduring spirit of the Burkinabé people.

CHAPTER 10
TOGO - EWE ELEGANCE

Welcome to the enchanting land of Togo, where the Ewe people's elegance and culinary finesse intertwine to create a unique gastronomic experience. In this chapter, we invite you to explore the flavors of Togo, where Ewe elegance celebrates the harmony between tradition, innovation, and the rich cultural heritage that defines this nation.

Discovering Togo's Ewe Culture

Togo, a nation known for its diverse ethnic groups, is deeply enriched by the traditions and creativity of the Ewe people. The flavors of Togolese cuisine reflect the influence of the Ewe people, who have preserved their cultural heritage through their distinct culinary artistry. From the bustling markets to the rural villages, Togolese culinary traditions honor both the past and the present.

Ewe Cuisine: A Symphony of Flavors

As you embark on your culinary journey through Togo, you'll encounter dishes that exemplify the elegance of Ewe cuisine. One such dish is akplε, a flavorful corn-based dumpling that embodies the creativity of the Ewe people in transforming simple ingredients into a culinary masterpiece. The Ewe people's mastery of akplε reflects their ability to blend tradition and innovation to create a dish that is both timeless and modern.

Akplε and the Art of Ewe Cooking

Akplε is more than just a dish; it's a symbol of the Ewe people's culinary craftsmanship. From its preparation to its presentation, akplε captures the essence of Ewe elegance. The way it's paired with soups, stews, and sauces showcases the way the Ewe people balance flavors to create a harmonious and exquisite dining experience.

Roots and Tubers: Ewe Staples

Togolese cuisine is anchored in the use of roots and tubers, reflecting the Ewe people's connection to the land and its offerings. Dishes like ablo, a steamed yam cake, and gboma dessert highlight the way the Ewe people transform these staples into dishes that celebrate both sustenance and flavor.

Seafood and the Gulf Influence

Togo's coastal location brings a bounty of seafood that plays a significant role in Ewe cuisine. The Ewe people's mastery of seafood preparation is evident in dishes like atike poisson, a grilled fish dish that reflects the Gulf of Guinea's influence on the culinary landscape. Seafood in Ewe cuisine is not just a meal; it's a testament to the Ewe people's relationship with the ocean and its treasures.

Ewe Sauces: A Flavorful Art Form

Sauces are at the heart of Togolese cuisine, and the Ewe people's creativity in preparing sauces is a testament to their culinary artistry. The use of ingredients like palm oil, groundnuts, and tomatoes in dishes like sauce feuilles demonstrates the way Ewe sauces elevate dishes to new heights, infusing them with depth, color, and flavor.

Ewe Festivals and Culinary Celebrations

In Togo, food is intrinsically tied to celebrations, festivals, and rituals that honor the cycles of life. The Ewe people's tradition of sharing meals during occasions like the Yam Festival showcases the role of food in fostering connections, celebrating traditions, and expressing gratitude. These culinary celebrations are a reflection of Togo's culture and the Ewe people's sense of belonging.

Culinary Heritage and Ewe Identity

Ewe cuisine is an embodiment of the Ewe people's cultural heritage, passed down through generations to preserve their identity and history. The way the Ewe people incorporate storytelling into their dishes, such as in the preparation of ablo, highlights the role of food in carrying forward traditions and narratives.

Ewe Spice and Elegance in Every Bite

Ewe cuisine is known for its delicate use of spices and herbs that enhance flavors without overpowering the senses. The way ingredients like ginger, garlic, and chili peppers are employed in dishes like atsi dokonu showcases the Ewe people's ability to create nuanced flavors that resonate on the palate.

The Art of Sharing: Ewe Community

Ewe culinary traditions are rooted in community and togetherness, reflecting the Ewe people's values of unity and harmony. The Ewe people's tradition of sharing meals with extended family and friends symbolizes the way food fosters connections, strengthens bonds, and creates moments of joy.

Ewe Elegance on Your Table

Throughout this chapter, you'll uncover a treasure trove of authentic Ewe recipes that embody the flavors and stories of Togo's culinary elegance. From akplε to atike poisson, each dish comes with step-by-step instructions and insights into the cultural significance behind it. By recreating these dishes in your own kitchen, you'll not only savor the richness of Togolese cuisine but also embrace the spirit of Ewe elegance, tradition, and community that these feasts symbolize.

Step into the world of Ewe elegance, where each recipe is an invitation to experience the flavors, traditions, and stories that shape Togo's vibrant culinary tapestry. As you savor the richness of Togolese cuisine, you'll be transported to the heart of the nation—a place where food is more than nourishment; it's a celebration of culture, a reflection of community, and a tribute to the enduring spirit of the Togolese people.

CONCLUSION
A SHARED CULINARY HERITAGE

As we bring our culinary expedition to a close, we find ourselves enriched by the vibrant flavors, diverse traditions, and shared stories that have unfolded across the landscapes of Africa. From the North African deserts to the West African coasts, from the savannas of Burkina Faso to the elegance of Togo, our journey has been a celebration of the rich tapestry of African cuisine. "A Shared Culinary Heritage" encapsulates the essence of our exploration, drawing together the threads of love, hope, betrayal, and culture that have woven their way through the chapters of this book.

Throughout our journey, one resounding theme has echoed across borders and tribes: the power of food to unite, to bridge differences, and to celebrate diversity. The act of breaking bread together is a universal language that transcends words, a gesture of fellowship that extends beyond cultural boundaries. We've witnessed how meals served in the heart of a home or shared at a communal feast become not only a source of nourishment but also a testament to the bonds that connect families, friends, and communities.

In the heart of each chapter, we discovered that the flavors of Africa are a result of intricate connections between history, environment, and the people who call this continent home. We witnessed how culinary traditions have been passed down through generations, carrying with them the stories of ancestors and the values that guide societies. Each recipe and dish is a reflection of resilience, innovation, and the ability of communities to adapt and transform humble ingredients into exquisite creations.

As we reflect on our journey, we recognize the moral lessons that have emerged from the stories told through food. We've learned that love and unity are constants that traverse cultural divides. Whether it's a newlywed couple sharing their first meal or a family gathering for a festival, the warmth of love and the spirit of togetherness are woven into every dish. We've witnessed the resilience of hope in the face of adversity, as communities turn scarcity into abundance and savor the joy that comes from sharing a meal. We've confronted the painful lessons of betrayal, understanding that the stories of individuals and societies are complex, reflecting both the light and shadow of human nature.

Culture, an intricate mosaic of beliefs, customs, and traditions, has been our guiding star on this culinary voyage. Through the flavors of Africa, we've seen culture come alive, honoring history and heritage while embracing the present. The recipes have offered more than just instructions for cooking; they've been a window into the values and spirit of each community, allowing us to glimpse the heart and soul of a people.

As we conclude our exploration, we are reminded that a shared culinary heritage is a tapestry of resilience, joy, and human connection. From the bustling markets to the quiet kitchens, from the feasts that fill the air with laughter to the simple meals that sustain families, food is more than sustenance; it's a celebration of life itself.

So, as you gather around the table to savor the dishes you've discovered in these pages, remember the stories that have been woven into every bite. Let each flavor be a reminder of the love that binds us, the hope that guides us, the betrayals that teach us, and the culture that enriches us.

ABOUT THE AUTHOR
'The Culinary Explorer'

Afful Christopher, the visionary author behind "West African Feasts - A Culinary Tapestry of Countries and Tribes," is a passionate culinary explorer driven by a love for culture, storytelling, and authentic flavors. With an unwavering fascination for West Africa's diverse cuisines and traditions, Afful embarked on a culinary journey to unearth the rich tapestry of tastes that define the region.

Fuelled by a lifelong appreciation for the way food connects people and communities, Afful's cookbook is a testament to meticulous research and a deep respect for culinary heritage. Every recipe is carefully crafted, reflecting not only the flavors but also the historical significance and cultural context of each dish. Afful's approach is immersive, born from genuine conversations with locals, market visits, and a profound understanding of the stories that ingredients carry.

9 7 9 8 8 6 0 0 6 9 5 4 1